AMAZAKE

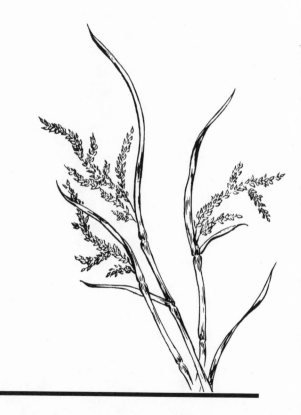

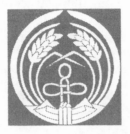

NATURALLY DELICIOUS & NUTRITIOUS

AMAZAKE

RICE BEVERAGE

John Finnegan
&
Kathy Cituk

CELESTIAL ARTS · BERKELEY, CALIFORNIA

A M A Z A K E

READER PLEASE NOTE: This book has been written solely for educational purposes. It should not be used as a substitute for advice of a physician or other medical practitioner. If you need medical treatment, you should seek out a medical practitioner. The authors provide this information with the understanding that you act on it at your own risk and with the full knowledge that you should consult with a health professional for any help you need.

CELESTIAL ARTS
P.O. Box 7327
Berkeley, California 94707

Cover and text design by Ken Scott
Word Processing by Hal Hershey
Drawings by Carol White
Typesetting by Ann Flanagan Typography

Library of Congress Cataloging-in-Publication Data

Finnegan, John, 1947-
   Amazake: naturally delicious, nutritious rice beverage /
John Finnegan
       p.   cm.
   "An Elysian Arts book."
   Includes bibliographical references.
   ISBN 0-89087-612-6
   1. Amazake.   I. Title.
TX412.F56   1990
641.8'77—dc20   90-35360
                                                          CIP

First Printing, 1990
0 9 8 7 6 5 4 3 2 1
94 93 92 91 90

Manufactured in the United States of America

ACKNOWLEDGEMENTS

This book is a creation of art and love from many people. Thanks to Ken Scott for the cover design and to Carol White for her drawings used throughout the book. To Tony Plotkin and Catherine Beu for all their time, information and help; and to Laurel Plotkin, Catherine Beu, Charles Kendall, and Elle Lockwood for their recipes.

—John Finnegan and
Kathy Cituk

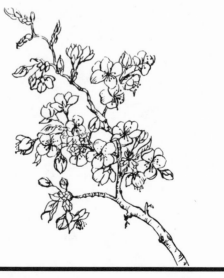

A M A Z A K E

CONTENTS

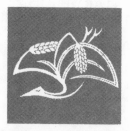

INTRODUCTION

Amazake is a delicious, refreshing drink made from whole grain brown rice. The rice is cooked, mixed with koji (a rice culture) or enzymes, then allowed to incubate for six to ten hours. The enzymes break down the complex starches in the rice into easily digestible, natural sugars. The resultant sweet liquid is high in fiber and B vitamins, low in fats, and contains no cholesterol.

Amazake is very versatile. It is great used as a dessert, snack, natural sweetening agent, or baby food, and can also be used to make kefir-yogurt, delicious smoothies, and tasty salad dressings. Frozen amazake makes excellent ice cream. Mix it with other ingredients to create luscious cookies, puddings, pies, and cakes.

This delicious beverage has no alcohol, preservatives or synthetic additives, and no added sugars or salts. It contains no dairy, wheat, or soy products, making it virtually nonallergic.

Amazake offers the superior nutritional benefits of brown rice. In this age of refined foods, it is a treat to discover this great-tasting whole food beverage.

1

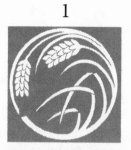

HISTORY & DEVELOPMENT

Most traditional cultures made some kinds of dessert beverages by fermenting grains or starchy vegetables. For hundreds of years the Japanese have made amazake, a delicious, nourishing drink from rice. This favorite beverage is served in restaurants and tea houses, and is also made in homes for special holiday celebrations. In the summer amazake is served cool, and in the winter it is served hot with grated ginger in it.

Amazake has been made in people's homes in the United States since the beginning of the 1900s. In 1978 Charles Kendall of Boston, Massachusetts, became the first person to produce this drink commercially in the United States. He made it on a small scale for several years, as a plain, high-quality, unfiltered drink. Today, Kendall produces a large amount of amazake, still using only organic grains and rice koji in its production.[1]

In 1981 Tony Plotkin of Grainaissance in Emeryville, California, developed a smooth, creamy amazake, added almond butter for flavoring—and the drink took off in popularity. He also developed a method of adding enzymes to largely replace the koji in breaking down the rice. This significantly reduced the cost of production. Under his creative direction, Grainaissance has grown to become the largest producer of amazake beverage in the Western hemisphere.

Many companies found innovative uses for amazake. Jean Poncé and Daniel Collin of Poncé Bakery in Chico, California, have developed a line of amazake pastries using the world's first oatmeal amazake, which they make themselves. Others have created amazake popsicles and puddings, and one of the biggest hits today is an amazake ice cream, called Rice Dream, produced by Imagine Foods in Palo Alto, California.

In 1983, in the *The Book of Miso*, William Shurtleff and Akiko Aoyagi forecast, "The first person to start commercial production of fine amazake in the West will, no doubt, receive eternal blessings of Heaven and Earth." With the development of such excellent products, we're sure all the companies will feel the blessings.

And the potential for public appreciation of this exceptionally fine quality beverage is great. As more and more people grow tired of getting poisoned from eating synthetic and processed foods, they are increasingly turning to products such as amazake, which tastes good and is nourishing as well.

As more people come to know about this unusual drink, amazake will, no doubt, make inroads into the supermarkets and maybe even vending machines. Grainaissance is currently marketing an aseptically packaged amazake which requires no refrigeration. Rice Dream Beverage is also available in aseptic packages.

1. Shurtleff, William and Akiko Aoyagi, *Amazake and Amazake Frozen Desserts: Industry and Market in North America* (Soy Foods Center, California, 1988).

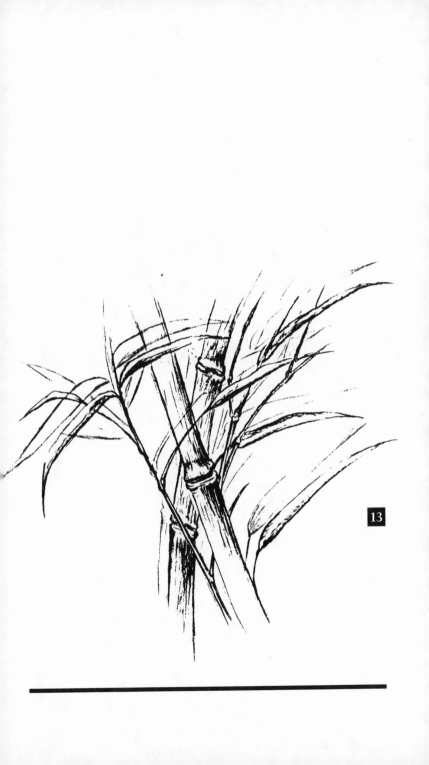

13

2

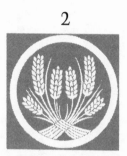

MAKING AMAZAKE

It is a little tricky to make amazake properly, but it can be done by using the following recipe provided by Tony Plotkin of Grainaissance.

---

1 cup uncooked
short grain brown rice
2 cups water
1 cup rice koji

(see "Sources for Amazake, Koji and Other Formulas")

Cook the rice with water as you would for table rice. Cool to 130 degrees. (It is very important to use a thermometer. The rice must be between 130 degrees and 135 degrees.) Transfer the rice to a bowl (stainless steel, glass, or ceramic). Mix koji into the rice and place the mixture in an incubator. Incubate at 130 degrees to 135 degrees for six to ten hours, stirring every three hours.

For incubation, you can use one of the following: 1) an oven, 2) a crock pot filled with water, set on low, with a bowl on top, or 3) a styrofoam ice chest with a heating pad in it. Keep the incubator within the exact temperature range or the koji may sour.

You now have amazake. Add 1½ cups water to the mixture, bring to a boil, and strain through a food mill to remove the bran. (The bran residue can be used in a muffin recipe.) Cool and flavor with fruit, spices, or nut butters.

DRINK.

3

COMPLEMENTARY FOODS, SPICES, & HERBS

Amazake is a sweet liquid. In traditional Eastern cooking and nutritional healing, its sweetness is often balanced with other foods or spices to increase wholesomeness. One of the best foods to combine with the amazake is almond butter. Almonds contribute protein, fatty acids, minerals, and vitamins, which greatly strengthen and balance amazake's nourishing properties. Soymilk is also an excellent complementary food, and when combined with amazake provides a complete protein. Fruit is also an excellent complement for amazake, especially bananas, peaches, apricots, raisins, and apples.

A little salt is also recommended. Among the spices and herbs, ginger and cinnamon are considered the most appropriate. Ginger warms and strengthens the stomach, digestive tract, and circulation. Cinnamon also warms and strengthens the system to balance the cooling, dispersing effects of desserts. These spices also purify the body, helping to prevent intestinal toxicity and proliferation of pathogenic organisms.

Kudzu, nutmeg, coriander, cardamom, and other tonifying herbs and spices are traditionally used to balance the sweetness of amazake. Kudzu thickens the amazake, which is helpful when making puddings and other desserts.

4

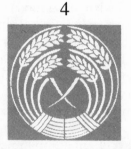

WHY USE
AMAZAKE?

Proper diet and nutrition are essential elements in maintaining or rebuilding good health. Unfortunately, in the United States, and increasingly around the world, convenience has become more important than nutrition. According to the U.S. Public Health Service Department, only 3,000,000 people out of the entire population can be considered healthy, about 1.5 percent.[1] This is not so surprising when you consider that the top ten sources of calories in the U.S. diet[2] are as follows:

1. White bread, rolls, crackers
2. Doughnuts, cookies, cakes
3. Alcoholic beverages
4. Whole milk
5. Hamburgers, cheeseburgers, etc.
6. Beef steaks, roasts
7. Soft drinks
8. Hot dogs, ham, lunch meat
9. Eggs
10. French fries, potato chips

The foods we eat are the building blocks our bodies use to create healthy organs and nervous systems, and keep them strong and functioning properly. The above list, however, does not provide much in the way of raw materials. Whole grains, beans, fish, poultry, fruits and vegetables are not even mentioned.

Nutritional deficiencies and poisons in our foods and environment are becoming major issues. Pesticides and industrial pollutants permeate our soil and water, poisoning the foods we eat. These poisons, along with the added preservatives and artificial flavoring and coloring agents, have been implicated as factors in causing cancer, heart disease, immune system breakdown, birth defects, mutations, sterility, and nervous system disorders.[3]

According to Samuel Epstein, M.D., in *The Politics of Cancer*, "The average American eats nine pounds of chemical additives a year, including preservatives, flavoring agents, stabilizers, and artificial colors. Therefore, over several decades of such dietary practice, the individual will have received several hundred pounds of food additives. Chemical agriculture and fast food industries are generating a whirlpool of artificial chemical elements which is making the modern diet increasingly inappropriate for human consumption."[4]

Not only do our foods contain many hidden poisons, the nutrients they provide have decreased significantly over the last few decades.[5] The lack of key enzymes, vitamins, minerals, protein, and fats in today's diets is a widespread and debilitating problem affecting the peoples of all industrialized nations. Many authorities feel that these deficiencies are causative factors in most disease, mental illness, and addictive behavior.

In December 1945 in the *United States Soil Conservation Publications*, the following statements were made:

"The U.S. produces more food than any other nation in the world. Yet, according to Dr. Thomas Parran, Jr., 40 percent of the population suffers from malnutrition." "...Evidently, the food eaten does not have enough of the right minerals and vitamins to keep them healthy.

"Investigators have found that food is no richer in nutrients than the soil from which it comes. Depleted soils will not produce healthy, nutritious plants. Plants suffering from mineral deficiencies will not nourish healthy animals. Mineral-deficient plants and under nourished animals will not support our people in health. Poor soils perpetuate poor people physically, mentally, and financially."[6]

The incidence of food and environmental allergies is also increasing, and many people today are allergic to dairy, wheat, or soy products. Amazake contains none of these, and is considered virtually nonallergic. It is also cholesterol free and low in fat and sodium.

The best way to create a strong, healthy body and mind is to live well and eat wholesome, unrefined foods prepared without poisonous ingredients and grown on good soils. Amazake, made from organic whole grain rice, provides the nourishment we need without the dangers of preservatives or added sugars, making it a good nutritional choice.

21

1. Hamaker, John, *The Survival of Civilization* (California: Hamaker-Weaver, 1982).
2. G. Block et al., 1985, *American Journal of Epidemiology*, 122:13-40.
3. Weissman, Joseph D., M.D., *Choose to Live: A Ten-Point, Ten-Week Program for Eliminating the Environmental Toxins That Threaten Your Health* (New York: Penguin Books, 1988).
4. Epstein, Samuel, M.D., *The Politics of Cancer* (Sierra Club, California, 1978).
5. Hamaker, op. cit.
6. Ibid.

5

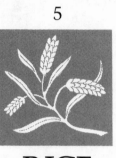

RICE

Rice is one of the most balanced, nourishing, and healing foods. It is soothing to the intestinal tract and easy to digest. It calms and stabilizes the nervous system, strengthens and regulates blood sugar, and builds strength, stamina, and muscle tissue. Those who are sensitive to dairy, wheat, or soy products find that they generally do not have an allergic reaction to rice. Rice is inexpensive, easy to cook, and lends itself to a wide variety of delicious dishes. Whole grain brown rice is also an excellent source of fiber, which is greatly deficient in today's diets.

Researchers are now discovering that remarkable substances such as gamma oryzanol and gamma frac are constituents of rice. These nutrients are being extracted from rice and used by physicians and nutritionists to build up muscle tissue and treat ulcers, nervous disorders, and other conditions.

Rice is well chosen as the basis of amazake. It is the staple food for more than one-half of the world's population and has been cultivated in the East for more than five thousand years. **Whole grain rice contains an excellent supply of vitamins, minerals, and carbohydrates, and, when combined with beans, nuts, seeds, or dairy products, forms a complete protein.**

One of the finest attributes of amazake is that through the action of the koji fermentation, and the enzymes, the rice is broken down, and all its nutrients are made available for easy assimilation. The complex carbohydrates are converted into the simple carbohydrates maltose and glucose. These simple carbohydrates, in combination with the grain's minerals, protein, vitamins, and fats, are very nourishing.

6

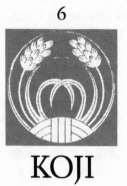

KOJI

Koji is a fermented product, usually made from rice or soybeans, that is used to ferment grains or beans to make foods such as miso, amazake, tempeh, tamari or shoyu, sake, pickles, and other products. **Koji is made from one of a select species of mold, usually a species of *aspergillus oryzae*.** These special molds are called koji starter. They have been carefully isolated from pathogenic molds, yeasts, and bacteria, and then cultivated for use in culturing food products, in the same way that acidophilus cultures are started.

The koji starter is then mixed into soybeans or rice or a similar grain and set to incubate in a warm place. The temperature is adjusted to different ranges throughout its process of fermentation, which takes several days. Making koji is a delicate and time-consuming operation. A good description of this process may be found in *The Book of Miso* by William Shurtleff and Akiko Aoyagi.

Koji can be purchased in large quantities from Miyako Oriental Foods, in both small and large quantities from Grainaissance, and from a few other suppliers as well. (See the Sources section on page 74 for the addresses of Grainaissance and Miyako Oriental Foods.)

7

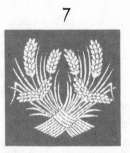

ALMOND AMAZAKE

The addition of almond butter to amazake was a stroke of sublime genius. Nutritionally, the almond provides a good amount of amino acids complementary to the amino acids in the amazake, producing a great-tasting drink with a substantial amount of complete protein. It also provides the key Omega 6 fatty acids and generous amounts of calcium, magnesium, phosphorus, potassium, riboflavin, and other important nutrients.

Edgar Cayce and many other nutritionists have long praised almonds, saying **they are the easiest of the nuts and seeds to digest, are the most alkaline, and have the best balance of minerals.** Historically they have been regarded as building strong bones and teeth.

8

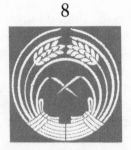

NUTRITIONAL ANALYSIS

Per 8-ounce serving

Adaptogens: Gamma oryzanol, gamma frac

Note: Nutritional analysis will vary according to type of rice used. Organic rice grown on good soils can contain as much as twice the protein and minerals of rice grown commercially on poor soils.

PLAIN AMAZAKE

Calories	210
Carbohydrates	49 g
Protein	5.5 g
Fat	1 g

Minerals:

Calcium	24 mg
Magnesium	64 mg
Potassium	157 mg
Sodium	6 mg
Zinc	1.4 mg
Iron	1.2 mg
Manganese	1.2 mg
Chromium	0 mg
Silica	0 mg
Selenium	29 mg
Phosphorus	162 mg
Copper	.15 mg

Vitamins:

B1	.26 mg
B2	.03 mg
B3	3.5 mg
B5	.79 mg
B6	.38 mg
B12	0 mg
A	0 mg
C	0 mg
D	0 mg
E	1.13 mg

ALMOND AMAZAKE

Calories	295
Carbohydrates	48 g
Protein	8.7 g
Fat	8 g

Minerals:

Calcium	51.7 mg
Magnesium	96 mg
Potassium	248.5 mg
Sodium	6.5 mg
Zinc	1.75 mg
Iron	1.76 mg
Manganese	1.43 mg
Chromium	0 mg
Silica	0 mg
Selenium	29.23 mg
Phosphorus	222 mg
Copper	.25 mg

Vitamins:

B1	.29 mg
B2	.14 mg
B3	3.51 mg
B5	.85 mg
B6	.39 mg
B12	0 mg
A	0 mg
C	0 mg
D	0 mg
E	1.8 mg

9

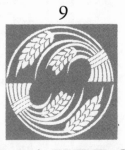

MAKERS
OF
AMAZAKE

KENDALL FOOD COMPANY

Charles Kendall was the first person to commercially produce amazake in North America, and he is still going strong. Kendall makes two flavors, plain and almond, and is one of the few companies to use the traditional method of preparing the amazake in earthenware crocks. The amazake contains organic brown rice, filtered water, sea salt and koji. No enzymes are used for the fermentation process.

Charles Kendall's favorite way to use amazake is to pour it over organic puffed rice for breakfast.

Kendall Food Company also produces mugwort mochi and natto.

GRAINAISSANCE

Grainaissance started as a producer of mochi in 1979. Two years later owner Tony Plotkin started making amazake. He was the first in the industry to introduce the use of enzymes in the process, which lowered the cost of the amazake and produced a creamier consistency. The bran was also filtered out, making the amazake even smoother, and almond butter was added to the ingredients, giving birth to the popular almond amazake shake. Unlike some amazake producers which use partially-milled brown rice, **Grainaissance uses only whole grain organic brown rice, yielding a beverage high in B vitamins and minerals with no cholesterol and low in fat.**

Grainaissance has continued to expand its amazake production and currently produces the following delicious flavors: Almond, Original (Plain), Mocha-Java, Apricot, and the new Coco-Almond and Vanilla Pecan.

Original and Almond flavors are also available in aseptic containers, which are lightweight and shelf stable, requiring no refrigeration before opening. Conveniently packaged with a straw, amazake is an ideal beverage to pack in lunches or take on hikes or picnics. And, since the aseptic package does not break easily and presents no cutting hazard to children, it is an ideal package for children to take to school and on field trips. Amazake can also be frozen right in the box for a delicious frozen treat.

Grainaissance also produces Soy Rice, a drink made from a combination of amazake, vanilla, and soy milk. It provides complete protein, and is a tasty milk substitute or snack. They also make mochi in Mugwort, Raisin-Cinnamon, Sesame-Garlic, and Regular flavors.

Amazake ingredients (Original flavor): water, whole grain organic brown rice, koji, enzymes.

IMAGINE FOODS
(Rice Dream)

Imagine Foods of Palo Alto started making amazake in 1982. Although moderately successful, amazake production was discontinued when the popular nondairy frozen dessert Rice Dream was developed in late 1984. **Today Rice Dream is the only naturally produced brown rice based frozen dessert in the marketplace.**

Like amazake, Rice Dream is made by a special enzyme process which converts the starches of cooked rice into its natural sugars. This produces a naturally sweet rice "milk" which is blended with unrefined oleic safflower oil, fresh fruit, vanilla, carob, or almonds, natural colors from annatto, turmeric, or beets, and vegetable stabilizers such as carob bean, guar seed and irish moss (carrageenan). The mixture is then put through an ice cream maker and frozen to produce the rich, creamy texture of Rice Dream.

No refined sugars are added. The natural sugars from the rice provide ample sweetness for the dessert, especially when combined with fruit and other flavors. The carob chips and fudge, however, do contain grain malts, but no white sugar, high fructose corn syrup, or honey is used.

This is one aspect that puts Rice Dream in a class by itself. Frozen soy, yogurt, and other dairy desserts are not naturally sweet, so sweeteners must be added to make them palatable. Rice

34

Dream also provides a virtually nonallergenic dessert for those who are sensitive to soy, dairy, or wheat products. And, unlike ice cream, it contains no cholesterol and is low in fat and calories.

Rice Dream is currently available in 13 flavors in pints, 2 flavors in quarts, and 3 flavors in bars; and Imagine Foods has plans to expand the line in the future.

Rice Dream Beverage in several flavors is also now available in shelf-stable aseptic packaging. The liquid version of Rice Dream is less sweet and thinner than other amazakes, providing a delicious, refreshing drink. It can be used as a milk substitute on cereal or in baking. The aseptic container makes it easy to take along on picnics and hikes, pack in school lunches for the kids, or take to work. No refrigeration is required.

Ingredients: Water, brown rice (partially milled), expeller pressed safflower oil, natural flavors, less than 3/10 of 1% of each of the following: lecithin, carob bean, guar gum, and carrageenan (from vegetable sources).

NUTRITIONAL INFORMATION:
VANILLA RICE DREAM
(4 oz. serving)

Calories	130
Carbohydrates	20 gm.
Fat	5 gm.
Cholesterol	0 gm.
Sodium	80 mg.

EDEN FOODS

Eden Foods has a longstanding reputation for providing high quality natural foods. Their product line includes the popular Edensoy soymilk, whole grains, whole grain cereals, flours, pastas, Japanese pastas, ramen, beans, cooking oils, vinegars, condiments, wholesome snacks, and a variety of traditional Japanese foods, including amazake, sea vegetables, and teas.

Eden Foods started importing organic amazake in 1982. It is produced in Japan by the traditional method, using organic whole grain brown rice. Eden amazake is packaged as a concentrated grain sweetener. It can be used as a leavener in breads and muffins, a substitute for refined sweeteners, a sweetener for hot cereals, or as a base for puddings, pies, and dairyless ice cream. It makes a thick, creamy milkshake when blended with fruit, soymilk, or water.

Eden Foods is probably best known for its best-selling Edensoy soymilk, which is a cholesterol-free, low sodium, non-dairy source of protein, iron, thiamine and phosphorus. Available in original, vanilla, and carob flavors, Edensoy is made from all organic ingredients and water purified with a reverse osmosis purification system. **It is a nutritious milk substitute for those who are sensitive to dairy products, and is available in the convenient aseptic package which requires no refrigeration until the package is opened.** Eden Foods was the first company to package soymilk in aseptic containers and is the largest producer of this popular beverage in North America.

SOOKE SOY FOODS LTD.

Grainwave is a line of health food products manufactured under the Canadian company name of Sooke Soy Foods Ltd. in Victoria, B.C. They currently make amazake in six flavors, mochi in six flavors, and vegetarian wheat cutlets in three flavors. They are distributed by all the major Canadian health food distributors.

The amazake (made from brown rice, water, and koji) is combined with fruits or nuts and is offered as a topping for desserts, pies, pancakes or cereals, as well as diluted for a creamy drink or frozen for a refreshing treat.

INFINITE FOODS

Infinite Foods of Philadelphia, Pennsylvania, started making amazake in 1982. They currently produce amazake in the following flavors: Banana, Chocolate, Almond, and Plain. They also make amazake puddings, seitan, and natto.

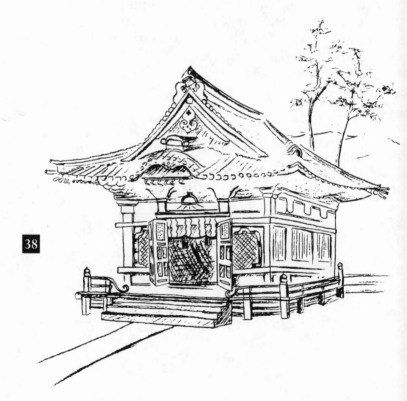

THE BRIDGE

The Bridge is a small company located in Middletown, Connecticut. They started making amazake in 1980 and currently produce a plain amazake using organic long grain brown rice and organic sweet rice. Sweet rice is the ingredient that distinguishes their amazake from the others. Koji is used, and no enzymes are added. The Bridge distributes amazake to Connecticut, Massachusetts, southern Vermont, West Chester County, NY, and New York City.

PONCÉ BAKERY

Although they do not distribute amazake, Poncé Bakery in Chico, California, has been making pastries with amazake since 1981. They make amazake out of oats rather than rice, which yields a thicker, protein-rich liquid that gives a sweet flavor and chewy texture to cakes, cookies, and other pastries. No refined sugars or preservatives are added, and all the ingredients are organic. The health conscious are glad to have such a delicious alternative to conventional baked goods.

The specialty of Poncé Bakery is bread. Flour is stone milled at the bakery, protecting the grain from damage caused by high-speed, high-heat processing. Bread is baked the same day, so flour does not have time to turn rancid. The bread is naturally leavened, so it holds its moisture longer than the rapidly-leavened bread produced by modern methods. Only organic ingredients are used.

Here's an unusual idea: Poncé Bakery offers a bread subscription club. Your prepaid subscription delivers your order to you when you want it. The subscription is a terrific gift idea—a certificate naming you as the benefactor is sent with the first loaf.

Ingredients (amazake cookies): organic whole oats, rice koji, organic almonds, organic raisins, water, sea salt.

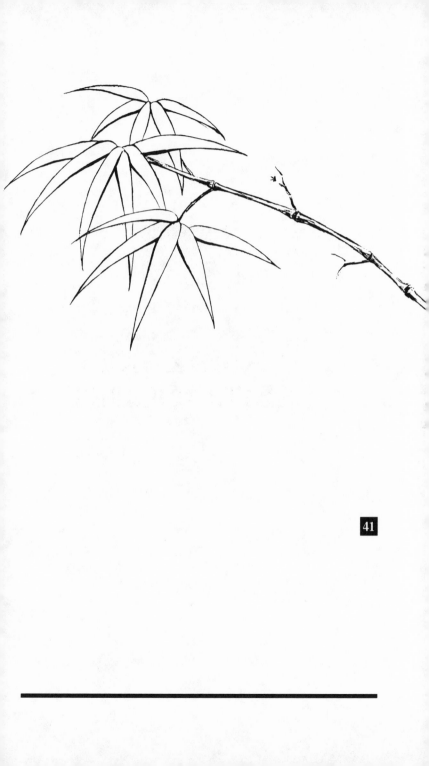

10

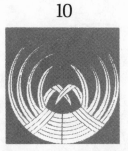

AMAZAKE
KEFIR-YOGURT

A complete colonization of the digestive tract with all the beneficial intestinal floras is essential to a healthy human body. A normal adult has three types of beneficial intestinal floras: *Streptococcus faecium*, acidophilus and bifidus. These bacteria are essential for human life. They help digest food, produce vitamins, and are a key factor in the body's control of pathogenic yeasts, bacteria, viruses, and parasites. They also appear to function in other ways that are important to the immune system but are as yet not completely understood.

Each of the three floras has distinct and critical functions, and an imbalance or deficiency in one can severely affect the functioning of the organism as a whole. For example, bifidus breaks down lactose, or milk sugar; a deficiency causes an inability to digest dairy products. In healthy infants, bifidus colonies make up 80 percent of their beneficial flora.

Abundant colonization of the digestive tract with these three floras is one of the main homeostatic mechanisms the body has for controlling the growth of and infection by pathogenic organisms. Proper colonization can be damaged by many things. The most common are stress, negative emotions, poor diet (lack of fiber and excessive consumption of refined foods and simple carbohydrates), and use of antibiotics, antiparasite medications, steroids, and birth control pills.

Incorporating a cultured amazake into your diet is an excellent and inexpensive way to build up your body's digestive floras. Culturing amazake with beneficial flora also increases its nutritional benefits. To make amazake kefir-yogurt, you follow the same procedure used to make yogurt from milk. Heat the amazake to 110 degrees, stirring constantly. Mix in 1 to 2 teaspoons of good-quality acidophilus or *Streptococcus faecium* floras, and incubate in a warm place (90 degrees to 120 degrees) for 24 hours. Since bifidus grows best in milk, it can be ingested separately. Any of the incubation methods discussed in Chapter 2 "Making Amazake" will work. This mixture will not gel as much as yogurt, but will yield a liquid similar to kefir. Some of the better brands of intestinal floras are: Jarrowdophilus, Sisudophilus, Maxidophilus, and others.

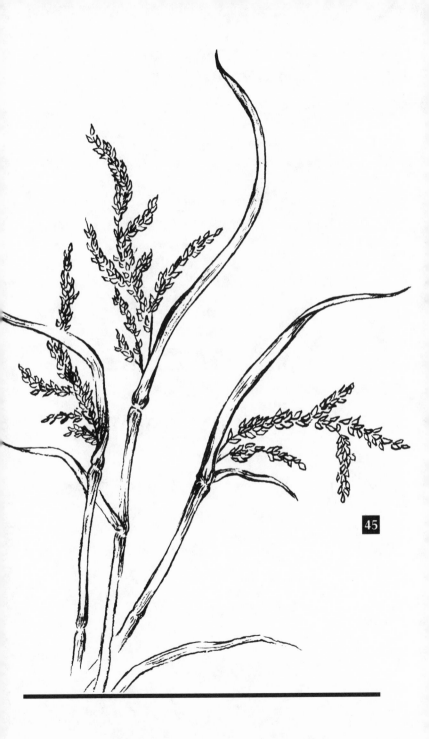

45

11

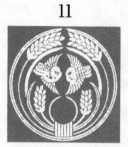

AMAZAKE
AS
BABY FOOD

One of the best uses for amazake is as baby food. Parents acclaim amazake, for in it they find a fine-tasting, all natural food containing most of the beneficial nutrients of whole grain brown rice, with fruit or almond butter added. The complex carbohydrates in the brown rice are converted into simple carbohydrates, making them easy to digest. In most amazakes some of the bran is removed.

Amazake is also economical. An eight-ounce serving costs about seventy-five cents, and diluted with two parts water for an infant food, it costs only about twenty-five cents for eight ounces, compared with fifty-three cents for eight ounces of leading baby foods. Parents often blend a little fresh or cooked fruit or cooked vegetables into the amazake to make a nourishing combination of baby foods.

Amazake can also be utilized during weaning from breast milk. It provides a naturally sweet, nourishing, soothing drink that is easily digested by babies and children. *It is not meant to be a substitute for mother's milk;* however, it is an excellent drink in between nursing or when the mother's milk is not plentiful enough to satisfy the baby. For babies six months old and younger, use one part amazake to two parts water. For babies older than six months, use one part amazake to one part water. Heat the amazake when diluting it with water; this helps the mixture to dissolve and taste much better.

Children who are sensitive to cow's milk or soy milk can use diluted amazake as a milk substitute. (However, amazake does not have the same nutritional content as cow's milk and should not be considered a complete milk substitute.)

It tastes great on its own, as well as poured over hot or cold cereals.

For nutritious baby foods, blend warm amazake with cooked fruit or vegetables. Try carrots, peas, broccoli, or zucchini. Also, try peaches, pears, bananas, strawberries, or apples. Be creative. The combinations are endless.

An important ingredient to include in a baby food is fresh bifidus. Bifidus bacteria are friendly bacteria that inhabit an infant's digestive tract and perform many functions essential to the infant's health and well-being. They help digest food, produce vitamins, help prevent excess toxins from forming in the gut, and are a key factor in the body's control of pathogenic yeasts, bacteria, viruses and parasites. They also appear to fulfill important but as yet not fully understood functions in maintaining a strong immune system.[1]

The last decade has shown a tremendous increase in the number of children with allergies, skin rashes, recurrent ear infections, and recurrent sinus and throat infections. Many of these problems have developed because the mothers' floras were destroyed through their use of antibiotics, antiparasite medications, birth control pills, or sometimes the excessive use of sugar, caffeine, or drugs.[2] These substances all destroy the beneficial digestive floras that the mother should pass on to her baby through nursing.[3]

An infant needs to be given generous, continual amounts of these floras from birth in order to prevent a yeast overgrowth in the digestive tract, which can indirectly cause many health problems. After beginning to take bifidus, these

48

symptoms usually show substantial improvement. Often they completely clear up in a matter of days. It is strongly recommended that bifidus be regularly included in the diets of all infants.

Bifidus is the best flora to give infants who are primarily milk fed, and acidophilus and *Streptococcus faecium* are the best floras to give infants and children who eat a primarily nonmilk diet. Mixing one-third teaspoon of good quality floras with amazake or milk will provide ample colonization of these essential creatures in infants' digestive tracts. Good brands are Lifestar, Ethical Nutrients, Metagenics, Sisudophilus, Jarrow-dophilus, Micro Flora, etc.

You can also make an excellent kefir-yogurt from amazake and feed this to infants and children to build up their digestive floras. (See the recipe on page 44 in this book.)

Also for infants, an excellent formula to mix with amazake is NuPlus. This unique herbal formula is produced by Sunrider International. A blend of extracted and concentrated Chinese herbs, it has excellent properties for building up strength and health. Mix one-half teaspoon in diluted Amazake and feed to the infant once or twice daily.

49

1. Finnegan, John, *Regeneration of Health* (California: Elysian Arts, 1987).
2. For an understanding of the influence of drugs in the creation of the yeast syndrome, see *Yeast Disorders* by John Finnegan, *The Yeast Syndrome* by John Trowbridge, M.D. and Morton Walker, D.P.M., and *The Yeast Connection* by William G. Crook, M.D.
3. Finnegan, John and Daphne Gray, *Recovery From Addiction* (California: Celestial Arts, 1990).

12

MILK
SUBSTITUTES

Commercial pasteurized milk today has residues of the pesticides, herbicides, antibiotics and hormones that the cows have ingested, and the vital enzymes and floras are destroyed in the pasteurization process. Amazake, used as a milk substitute, has none of the drawbacks of commercial, pasteurized milk. When diluted with water, it can be used as a milk substitute for drinking, cooking and baking. Use two parts plain amazake to one part water for a nonfat or lowfat milk substitute. Two parts almond amazake to one part water yields a good substitute for whole milk, because it contains protein, minerals, vitamins, and the unrefined oil from the almond butter. **For a complete protein, combine amazake, soy milk, and water to taste, or use almond amazake.**

Amazake can also be substituted for cream or milk to thicken soups such as split pea, cream of broccoli, cream of asparagus, or corn chowder.

13

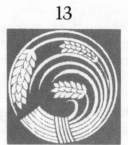

THE
FUTURE
OF
AMAZAKE

Consumers are becoming more and more conscious of what they eat. Recognition is growing that diet plays a key role in health and well-being and that wholesome, natural foods are the best source of nutrition. **More and more people are turning to natural foods to replace refined and fast foods.**

Amazake has tremendous potential as a viable, delicious alternative to milkshakes and soft drinks, which often contain sugar, caffeine, propylene glycol (antifreeze), artificial colors, and artificial flavors.

Frozen amazake, which contains no added sugar or preservatives, provides a nutritious alternative to commercial ice creams, which are often made with toxic substances mentioned above.

Aseptic packaging makes it possible for amazake to be stocked in grocery and convenience stores, and it can even be available in vending machines in airports, shopping malls, office buildings—anywhere. Someday maybe restaurants will recognize the potential and begin to offer amazake on their menus. Imagine having a healthy, delicious, natural drink and snack as available as the popular soft drinks and fast foods!

14

RECIPES

ZESTY AMAZAKE
SALAD DRESSING
(from Grainaissance)

1 cup plain amazake
½ cup mayonnaise
2 tablespoons vinegar
1 tablespoon red or white miso
1 clove garlic

Mix all ingredients in blender and dress up your favorite salad.

WARM GINGER
AMAZAKE
(from Grainaissance)

1 cup plain amazake
¾ cup water
¼ to ½ teaspoon grated ginger

Bring amazake and water to a boil. Remove from heat and stir in ginger. Serve in tea cups for a cozy after dinner drink. This is a traditional Japanese drink that is very soothing. Serves two.

　　Note: It is common to dilute amazake in a variety of ways, such as this recipe. For a variation of this recipe, try heating the almond amazake diluted with water. It'll remind you of morning cocoa.

PANCAKES
(from Elle Lockwood)

1 cup whole wheat flour
1 cup rye, blue corn, or oat flour
½ to ¾ cup canola or safflower oil
1 cup amazake
1 teaspoon baking soda
2 teaspoons baking powder
1 teaspoon vanilla extract
½ to 1 teaspoon cinnamon

Mix ingredients together in a bowl, making sure batter is not too thick. Drop batter onto hot griddle, and cook until golden brown. Makes six.

FRENCH TOAST

1 egg
3 tablespoons amazake
¼ teaspoon vanilla extract
Dash cinnamon

Mix ingredients with a fork. Soak bread in mixture and cook in butter in a heavy skillet. Delicious! Serves two.

AMAZAKE
EGG NOG
(from Grainaissance)

8 ounces plain amazake
8 ounces almond amazake
1 teaspoon vegetable oil (optional)
2 egg yolks (optional)
1 pinch cinnamon
1 pinch sea salt
¼ teaspoon natural vanilla flavoring
¼ teaspoon natural rum flavor (optional)
1 pinch turmeric (for color) or
  annatto (if you can find it)
1 pinch fresh crushed nutmeg
  (very important)

Mix all ingredients together in a blender.
Makes one quart.

CHESTNUT CREAM PIE
(from Grainwave)

3 cups amazake
1½ cups chestnuts, boiled and peeled
2 tablespoons tahini, roasted
1 tablespoon agar flakes
1 tablespoon kudzu dissolved in
   3 tablespoons water
⅓ cup rice syrup
¼ teaspoon sea salt
1 tablespoon vanilla
1 teaspoon lemon juice
1 pie crust

Heat amazake and agar flakes for 10 minutes.
Stir in kudzu. Bring to a boil. Add rice syrup and
vanilla. Place mixture in blender or cuisinart with
chestnuts, tahini, and lemon juice. Blend until
smooth. Pour into pie crust. Chill and serve.

AMAZAKE COOKIES

(from Eden Foods)

1 package Eden Amazake
⅓ cup barley malt or sorghum molasses
½ cup corn oil
1 teaspoon vanilla
½ cup apple juice or Original or
    Vanilla Edensoy soymilk
½ teaspoon sea salt
4 cups whole wheat pastry flour
Eden Mirin for optional glaze

Mix all liquid ingredients in a bowl. Add seasonings for desired cookie variation. Add salt and flour, 1 cup at a time, stirring vigorously after each addition. Dough will be quite soft. Roll in waxed paper and chill for at least 4 hours.

When thoroughly chilled, roll out ¼-inch thick on a floured surface and cut into desired shapes. To assure dough stays chilled, work with ⅓ of the dough at a time, keeping the balance in the refrigerator. Bake for 15 to 20 minutes in a 375 degree oven. Glaze by brushing on mirin with a pastry brush 5 minutes before cookies are done.

VARIATIONS:

GINGERBREAD MEN

Add:
¼ teaspoon ground cloves
½ teaspoon ground cinnamon
2–3 teaspoons freshly grated ginger

Cut into gingerbread men shapes and decorate with raisins for eyes and buttons.

COOKIE TARTS

Cut into round shapes and make indentation with thumb. Fill with Eden Apple Butter.

LEMON NUT DROPS

Add:
1 tablespoon grated lemon peel
3 tablespoons lemon juice
¾ cup chopped roasted walnuts or pecans

60

BRANDY SNAPS

Add:
¼ teaspoon freshly grated ginger
½ teaspoon each of cinnamon,
   grated lemon, and orange rind
2–3 teaspoons of brandy

FROZEN DESSERT TREATS

These dessert treats are both nutritious and delicious. Kids love them and parents can serve them without worrying about added sugars, preservatives, or refined foods. Amazake makes a great "ice cream." Just put it in a container that has a large enough opening to be able to be scooped out, and freeze. Be sure to leave some room at the top, as amazake expands as it freezes. Amazake can also be frozen in the aseptic box. When the box is cut open, the frozen Amazake can be squeezed up and eaten—a great on-the-go treat!

AMAZAKE POPSICLES
(from Grainaissance)

1 to 2 cups any flavor of amazake

Fill a popsicle maker with amazake and freeze. Almond amazake popsicles are a favorite with many people. A great refreshment for a warm day.

AMAZAKE FRUIT MILKSHAKE

4 ounces any flavor amazake
4 ounces water
2 scoops frozen amazake
Frozen strawberries or other frozen fruit

Mix amazake, water, and frozen fruit thoroughly in a blender. Add the frozen amazake and mix slightly for a refreshing, delicious shake. Serves one.

MOCHA-JAVA MILKSHAKE

4 ounces mocha-java amazake
4 ounces water
2 scoops frozen mocha-java amazake

Mix amazake and water thoroughly in a blender. Add the frozen amazake and mix slightly. For those of us who love the taste of coffee, but don't like the caffeine! Serves one.

AMAZAKE SUNDAES

3 scoops frozen amazake
Strawberries, crushed pineapple,
    chocolate sauce, bananas, chopped nuts

Choose your favorite flavor of frozen amazake, and then be creative with your favorite toppings! Serves one.

AMAZAKE FLOATS

Add two scoops of frozen amazake to natural
ginger ale, root beer or cola. Delicious! Serves one.

AMAZAKE FRUIT JUICE
SPARKLERS

Add two scoops of frozen amazake to your favorite
fruit juice and sparkling water. Sparkling!
Serves one.

AMAZAKE GELATIN DESSERT
(from Grainaissance)

1 cup amazake
  (almond, mocha-java or apricot)
1 tablespoon agar-agar flakes
  (sea vegetable gelatin)

Add agar-agar to amazake. Stir and bring to a boil.
Reduce heat and simmer five minutes or until
dissolved. Pour into a bowl and chill until firm.
Serves two.

CAROB
AMAZAKE FROSTING
(from Grainaissance)

1 tablespoon kudzu starch (or cornstarch)
1 cup plain amazake
¼ cup unsweetened carob chips
¼ teaspoon vanilla

Dissolve kudzu starch in amazake. Stir continuously and bring to a boil. Reduce heat and simmer for one hour, stirring occasionally. Then stir in carob chips and vanilla, and cool. Now frost your favorite cake. Makes ¾ cup.

VANILLA
AMAZAKE PUDDING
(from Catherine Beu)

1 pint plain amazake
3 tablespoons kudzu or arrowroot
  (1½ tablespoons per cup amazake)
1 teaspoon vanilla
¼ teaspoon ginger juice or
  powdered ginger
¼ teaspoon nutmeg or coriander (optional)

Dilute the kudzu or arrowroot in the smallest amount of water possible. When completely dissolved, add to the amazake and slowly bring the mixture to a boil, stirring constantly. One or two minutes after the mixture thickens completely, turn off the heat. Cool several minutes and add vanilla, ginger, and other spices. (To make the ginger juice, grate fresh ginger on the fine part of a grater. Squeeze the juice out of the pulp into a cup.) Mix spices in well. Chill pudding or eat warm. Serves four.

VARIATIONS :

ALMOND
AMAZAKE PUDDING

Follow the preceding recipe, but use almond amazake and leave out nutmeg and coriander.

MOCHA-JAVA
AMAZAKE PUDDING

Follow the preceding recipe, but use mocha-java amazake and leave out ginger and spices.

APRICOT
AMAZAKE PUDDING

Follow the preceding recipe, but use apricot amazake and leave out ginger and spices. Soak dried organic apricots in apricot amazake or water, and then proceed with recipe. Try it smooth too!

Note: When making pudding, some amazakes need to be brought to a boil and cooked for ten minutes before adding starch, or the enzyme content can prevent the pudding from setting.

OATMEAL COOKIES

(from Catherine Beu)

1 tablespoon ground sesame seeds (no salt)
1½ cups rolled oats
1½ cups organic whole wheat pastry flour
¼ teaspoon sea salt
1 tablespoon lecithin granules
2 tablespoons corn oil
1 teaspoon vanilla
¾ cup barley malt or rice syrup
1 cup amazake (makes cookies rise!)
¾ cup raisins and ½ cup chopped walnuts

Combine first five dry ingredients. Fluff them lightly together with a fork. (Add raisins and walnuts *after* wet ingredients.) Combine wet ingredients together and slowly add to dry ingredients. Now add raisins and walnuts. Let sit one-half hour or longer in a warm place. Form into cookies and place on a cookie sheet greased with corn or sesame oil. Bake at 350 degrees until golden brown. (This could take 15, 20, or 30 minutes, depending on your oven.) Enjoy! Makes one dozen.

BAKING WITH AMAZAKE: When you use amazake as an ingredient for cakes and cookies, be aware that amazake is a very mild sweetener. To achieve the sweetness of traditional cakes and cookies, you need to add some other sweetener such as honey, maple syrup, or barley malt, along with amazake. A noticeable feature of baking with amazake is the delicious, moist texture it gives baked goods.

AMAZAKE SMOOTHIES

CREAMY BANANA-SESAME DRINK
(from Grainaissance)

1 cup plain amazake
1 tablespoon sesame tahini
1 ripe banana
½ cup water

Mix ingredients together in a blender. This is a pleasantly satisfying drink. Serves one.

SMOOTHIE

6 ounces water or herbal tea
6 ounces amazake
1 teaspoon to 2 tablespoons bee pollen
1 teaspoon flax seed oil
2 tablespoons nutritional yeast (optional)
1 teaspoon unpasteurized white miso
1 to 2 tablespoons NuPlus

Mix ingredients together in a blender. Serves one.

BODY BUILDING
SMOOTHIE SUPREME

5 ounces almond amazake
5 ounces water or herbal tea
1 teaspoon to 2 tablespoons bee pollen
1 teaspoon flax seed oil
1 to 2 tablespoons NuPlus
½ teaspoon acidophilus powder
1 raw egg yolk

Mix ingredients together in a blender. Serves one.

ULTIMATE HEALTH
AND BODY BUILDING SMOOTHIE

6 ounces water or herbal tea
6 ounces amazake
1 tablespoon bee pollen
1 to 2 tablespoons NuPlus
6 capsules Korean Ginseng*
½ teaspoon acidophilus powder
1 teaspoon flax seed oil
1 raw egg yolk

Mix ingredients together in a blender. Serves one.
*Note: Empty powder from capsules.

ABOUT THE INGREDIENTS

NUTRITIONAL YEAST

Yeast is a tremendous food supplement. It provides high amounts of all the B vitamins, protein, potassium, zinc, RNA, and other key nutrients. Some brands have much higher amounts of nutrients and taste much better than others. Kal is an excellent brand.

EGG YOLKS

Raw egg yolks are a good source of many important nutrients that strengthen and regenerate the endocrine glands, liver, nervous system, and immune system. Many Eastern sages recommend eating raw egg yolk every day to strengthen the entire system. Dr. Henry Bieler recommended that those with nervous system and adrenal collapse eat several raw egg yolks daily to rebuild their health.[1]

FLAX SEED OIL

According to many authorities, the most widespread nutritional deficiency today is oxygen, and the second and third most deficient nutrients are the Omega 3 and Omega 6 fatty acids. These key nutrients play a vital part in most of the main functions of the body. They are essential to the transportation of oxygen, the functioning of the immune system, the production of energy, and the integrity and strength of the cell membranes. They also provide the raw materials for the body to build many of its key hormones.[2]

MISO

Miso is made from fermented soybeans which are usually combined with barley or other grains. It is a delicious addition to soups and salad dressings, providing easily digested complete protein. Unpasteurized miso is acclaimed for its ability to aid in digestion and assimilation of other foods. Miso comes in a variety of flavors, which vary in salt content, and bring out the flavor and nutritional value in foods. The oils contained in miso give it its savory flavor and aroma, and aid in dispersing accumulations of cholesterol and other fatty acids in the circulatory system.

A major study conducted in Japan found that those who drank miso soup every day had 32 to 33 percent less stomach cancer than those who did not drink it. In Japan, it is believed that miso promotes long life and good health, can cure colds, improve metabolism, clear the skin, and help resist parasitic diseases. It is also used to settle an upset stomach and get rid of a hangover. Miso has been found to contain dipicolinic acid, which attaches to radioactive metals and discharges them from the body. Some people have found that taking miso soup every day helps to alleviate the side effects of radiation therapy. It has also been found to neutralize some of the effects of smoking and air pollution.[3]

70

BEE POLLEN

Bee pollen is one of mankind's oldest and most widely used nutritional and rejuvenating formulas.

It is the only food that has all the protein, vitamins, minerals, fats, and carbohydrates necessary to sustain life. It has also been found to contain special nutrients that strengthen the metabolism, endocrine glandular, and immune system functions. A large number of medical studies have been done showing its efficacy for fatigue, weakness, allergies, colds, neurasthenia, prostatitis, arthritis, and general degenerative conditions.

Each individual pollen granule is contained within a hard shell that resists digestion. Two companies (High Desert Pollen and 3rd Day Botanicals) have developed methods to fracture the hard exterior shell and make the vital inner nutrients available. A small percentage of people are allergic to pollen, but most can use it safely.

SUNRIDER
CHINESE HERBAL FORMULAS

Sunrider Chinese herbal formulas are based on unique herbal combinations developed thousands of years ago by Shaolin sages. Grown mostly on organic soils, extracted, and concentrated up to eight times, these herbal formulas nourish and strengthen body systems. These are tonic food herbs as opposed to medicinal herbs, so they can be taken every day to increase strength and health without creating an imbalance.

71

1. Bieler, Henry, *Food Is Your Best Medicine* (New York: Vintage, 1973).
2. Rudin, Donald O., M.D., and Felix, Clara, *The Omega 3 Phenomenon* (New York: Rawson Associates, 1987) and Gittleman, Ann Louise, M.S., *Beyond Pritikin* (New York: Bantam, 1988).
3. Shurtleff, William, and Akiko Aoyagi, *The Book of Miso* (California: Ten Speed Press, 1983).

APPENDIX I:

ABOUT ASEPTIC PACKAGING

Awareness of the environmental impact of food processing and packaging is growing. Concerned people everywhere are examining more closely the techniques and materials used, especially for packaging.

Aseptic packaging is a multi-layer laminate, composed of paper (over 70%) bonded to thin layers of polyethylene and aluminum foil. The aluminum layer is extremely thin (.0036 inch) and weighs less than 1/20th of an ounce. The contents of the package never come into contact with the aluminum. In the aseptic containers used by Grainaissance, Imagine Foods, and Eden Foods, the paper layers are not bleached or treated with dioxin, and the ink on the outside is water soluble and contains no heavy metals. The polyethylene used in the laminate is made from pure, additive-free virgin resin. Each shipment of packaging material is tested for the migration of polyethylene before it is sold.

There are numerous advantages to using aseptic packaging. Beverages protected in aseptic packages do not need to be refrigerated before opening, and the package provides a complete barrier to light, air, and bacteria. Since the package does not break easily and is made mostly of paper, it is safe for even small children to use, without the cutting hazard that glass bottles and aluminum cans present.

Although it is not biodegradable, it is considered very "environmentally friendly." Aseptic packages can be recycled. A plant is being built in West Germany to build particle board from used aseptic packages. In Canada, used aseptic packages will be used as raw material for making plastic composite lumber. The new material will be water-proof and maintenance-free, and will be used for park benches, sign posts, picnic tables, and similar objects. Environmentally clean compost, or top-soil, has also been made with aseptic packages.

Aseptic packages actually burn cleaner than fossil fuels. Much of the energy contained in the package can be recovered by incineration. If the aseptic package is burned at a high temperature in a municipal incinerator even the aluminum burns and yields energy. The end product is aluminum oxide, one of its naturally occurring forms in nature.

Replacing glass bottles in landfills with asep-tic packages would reduce the volume of waste substantially. Also, not requiring refrigeration uses less electricity and reduces CFC's (chloro-fluorocarbons) which damage the ozone layer. The space-saving square shape of the aseptic package uses both less material and less storage space. In a truckload of bottled beverages, 70% of the load is food and 30% is packaging. For aseptic, 90% is food and 10% is packaging. Transportation costs are significantly reduced, resulting in less air pollution.

The number of companies using aseptic pack-aging for their products is increasing. Eden Foods, Grainaissance, and Imagine Foods are ecologi-cally-minded companies currently using this smart packaging.

Source: *Edensoy, Aseptic Packaging and the Environment* (Michigan: Eden Foods, Inc., 1990).

APPENDIX II:

SOURCES FOR AMAZAKE AND KOJI

If you wish to try amazake you can probably find it in your local natural foods or grocery store. If your store doesn't carry it, a store employee can order it. Below is a list of companies that are currently producing or importing amazake:

GRAINAISSANCE
1580 62nd Street
Emeryville, CA 94608
(415) 547-7256

EDEN FOODS, INC.
701 Tecumseh Road
Clinton, MI 49236
(517) 456-7424
(800) 248-0301

IMAGINE FOODS, INC.
299 California Avenue
Suite 305
Palo Alto, CA 94306
(415) 327-1444

INFINITE FOODS
1872 East Schiller Street
Philadelphia, PA 19134
(215) 739-8578

KENDALL FOOD COMPANY
46A Route 112
Worthington, MA 01098
(413) 238-5928

SOOKE SOY FOODS, LTD.
4247 Dieppe Road
Victoria, B.C.
Canada V8X 2N2
(604) 479-4088

THE BRIDGE
598 Washington Street
Middletown,CT 06457
(203) 346-3663

Amazake pastries can be purchased from:

PONCÉ BAKERY
116 West 12 Street
Chico, CA 95928
(916) 891-8354

Koji can be purchased from the following:

GRAINAISSANCE
1580 62nd Street
Emeryville, CA 94608
(415) 547-7256

MIYAKO ORIENTAL FOODS
4287 Puente Avenue
Baldwin Park, CA 91706
(818) 962-9633

Other sources for koji and koji starter can be found in *The Book of Miso* by William Shurtleff and Akiko Aoyagi.

BIBLIOGRAPHY

Aihara, Herman, *Basic Macrobiotics*, New York: Japan Publications, 1985

Bieler, Henry, *Food Is Your Best Medicine*, New York: Vintage, 1973

Chishti, Hakim, N.D., *The Traditional Healer*, Vermont: Healing Arts Press, 1988

Esko, Edward & Wendy, *Macrobiotic Cooking For Everyone*, New York: Japan Publications, 1980

Finnegan, John, *Regeneration of Health*, California: Elysian Arts, 1987

Finnegan, John, *Yeast Disorders*, California: Elysian Arts, 1987

Finnegan, John, *Understanding Oils and Fats*, California: Elysian Arts, 1990

Gittleman, Ann Louise, M.S., *Beyond Pritikin*, New York: Bantam, 1988

Grow Company, *Scientific Comparative Studies and Bioavailability Studies on U.S.P. Minerals and Grow Company Minerals*, California: Lifestar, 1986

Grow Company, *Scientific Comparative Studies and Bioavailability Studies on U.S.P. Vitamins and Grow Company Re-Natured Vitamins*, California: Lifestar, 1986

Hamaker, John, *The Survival of Civilization*, California: Hamaker-Weaver Publishers, 1982

Kirschmann, John, *Nutrition Almanac*, New York: McGraw-Hill, 1984

Lu, Henry, *Chinese System of Food Cures*, New York: Sterling Co., 1986

Rodale, J.I. and Staff, *Complete Book of Minerals For Health*, Pennsylvania: Rodale Books

Rudin, Donald O., M.D., and Felix, Clara, *The Omega 3 Phenomenon*, New York: Rawson Associates, 1987.

Shurtleff, William, and Akiko Aoyagi, *The Book of Miso*, California: Ten Speed Press, 1983

Shurtleff, William, and Akiko Aoyagi, *Amazake: Industry Study*, California: Soy Foods Center, 1988

Teegarden, Ron, *Chinese Tonic Herbs*, New York: Japan Publications, 1985

Tierra, Michael, N.D., *The Way Of Herbs*, New York: Pocket Books, 1983

Articles
East / West Journal, June, 1990, Jan Belleme.

GLOSSARY

acidophilus—one of the three major beneficial intestinal floras found in the digestive tracts of healthy human beings. See "Amazake Kefir-Yogurt" page 44.

aseptic package—see Appendix I "About Aseptic Packaging"

bifidus—one of the three major beneficial intestinal floras found in the digestive tracts of healthy human beings. See "Amazake Kefir-Yogurt" page 44.

enzymes—catalysts for conversion of carbohydrates. Enzymes are used in the production of amazake to break down the complex carbohydrates of the rice into simple carbohydrates (sugars).

kefir-yogurt—the thick, semisolid food made from the cultured milk or amazake. See "Amazake Kefir-Yogurt" page 44.

koji—rice cultured with *Aspergillus oryzae* mold. This culture is then added to cooked rice, and the mixture is allowed to ferment for several hours to form amazake.

mochi—a traditional Japanese food made from steamed and pounded glutinous (sweet) brown rice. It is packaged in flat squares which puff up when baked in the oven. It comes in a variety of flavors including plain, mugwort, raisin-cinnamon, and sesame-garlic.

miso—a fermented soybean paste used as a base for soups, salad dressings, and other dishes. See "miso" page 68.

mugwort—a green herb rich in iron and calcium. It is known to help make hemoglobin for healthy blood, and has traditionally been eaten by people with anemia and pregnant and breast-feeding women to aid their developing infant. It is an ingredient in mochi.

natto—fermented soybean product.

seitan—a "wheat cutlet" made from the gluten of whole wheat, shoyu, herbs and spices, and seaweed. It is a good source of protein and is often used as a vegetarian substitute for meat.

streptococcus faecium—one of the three major beneficial intestinal floras found in the digestive tracts of healthy human beings. See "Amazake Kefir-Yogurt" page 44.

ABOUT THE AUTHORS

John Finnegan was born in Greenwich Village and raised in Long Island, the jungles of Latin America, and the beaches and redwoods of Northern California. He began writing his first book when he was nine years old—the story of his family's journey from New York to Lima, Peru. They were the first people to drive the length of Central America, often having to cut their own road through the jungle with machetes, shovels, and pickaxes.

At nineteen, he began to research the biochemical basis of physical and mental illness, which included studying and working with many of this century's leading medical pioneers. He studied life sciences and social sciences at San Francisco State University, College of Marin, and continued his studies with Dr. John Christopher, Dr. Michael Barnett, Piro Caro, other holistic researchers, and in several medical centers. John Finnegan is the author of six books, including *Recovery From Addiction*, which he co-authored with Daphne Gray. He lectures and conducts seminars, and gave presentations at both the 1987 and 1988 San Francisco Whole Life Expos.

Kathy Cituk has traveled in South America, Europe, the Middle East, and India, and appreciates the cuisines of many cultures. She has edited several books on health and nutrition and co-authored *Natural Foods and Good Cooking* with John Finnegan. She enjoys the peaceful solitude of the woods and beaches along the California coast where she resides.